# 海南出入境游艇检疫管理办法

Administrative Measures on Quarantine of Entry-Exit Yachts of Hainan Province

中国质检出版社
中国标准出版社
CHINA ZHIJIAN PUBLISHING HOUSE
STANDARDS PRESS OF CHINA
北 京
BEIJING

图书在版编目(CIP)数据

海南出入境游艇检疫管理办法＝Administrative Measures on Quarantine of Entry-Exit Yachts of Hainan Province：汉英对照/国家质检总局法规司,国家质检总局标准法规中心编译．—北京：中国标准出版社,2014.1

ISBN 978-7-5066-7429-4

Ⅰ.①海… Ⅱ.①国… Ⅲ.①游艇—国境检疫—卫生检疫—海南省 Ⅳ.①R185.3

中国版本图书馆 CIP 数据核字(2013)第 300447 号

中国质检出版社
中国标准出版社　出版发行
北京市朝阳区和平里西街甲 2 号(100013)
北京市西城区三里河北街 16 号(100045)
网址 www.spc.net.cn
总编室:(010)64275323　发行中心:(010)51780235
读者服务部:(010)68523946
中国标准出版社秦皇岛印刷厂印刷
各地新华书店经销

\*

开本 880×1230　1/32　印张 1.5　字数 23 千字
2014 年 1 月第一版　2014 年 1 月第一次印刷

\*

定价:**10.00** 元

如有印装差错　由本社发行中心调换
版权专有　侵权必究
举报电话:(010)68510107

# 目 录

中华人民共和国国家质量监督检验检疫总局令
（2013 年第 153 号）………………………… 1

海南出入境游艇检疫管理办法 ……………… 3
    第一章    总则 ………………………………… 3
    第二章    入境检疫 …………………………… 4
    第三章    出境检疫 …………………………… 8
    第四章    监督管理 …………………………… 8
    第五章    法律责任 …………………………… 10
    第六章    附则 ………………………………… 12

# 中华人民共和国
# 国家质量监督检验检疫总局令

**第 153 号**

《海南出入境游艇检疫管理办法》已经 2013 年 4 月 23 日国家质量监督检验检疫总局局务会议审议通过，现予公布，自 2013 年 8 月 1 日起施行。

局长

2013 年 6 月 5 日

# 海南出入境游艇检疫管理办法

## 第一章 总 则

**第一条** 为防止疫病疫情传入传出,规范海南出入境游艇检疫,根据《中华人民共和国国境卫生检疫法》及其实施细则、《中华人民共和国进出境动植物检疫法》及其实施条例、《国际卫生条例》等法律法规和国务院有关规定,制定本办法。

**第二条** 本办法适用于从海南出境、入境游艇的检疫和监督管理工作。

**第三条** 国家质量监督检验检疫总局(以下简称国家质检总局)主管全国出入境游艇检疫监督管理工作。

国家质检总局设在海南的出入境检验检疫机构(以下简称检验检疫机构),负责海南出入境游艇检疫和监督管理工作。

**第四条** 海南出入境游艇检疫监督管理遵循先行先试、监管有效、简化手续、方便快捷的原则。

## 第二章 入境检疫

**第五条** 入境游艇必须在最先抵达的口岸接受检疫。

检验检疫机构可以对入境游艇实施电讯检疫、锚地检疫、靠泊检疫或者随船检疫。

**第六条** 艇方或者其代理人应当在游艇抵达口岸前，向入境口岸检验检疫机构申报下列事项：

（一）游艇名称、国籍、预定抵达检疫地点的日期和时间；

（二）发航港、最后寄港；

（三）游艇操作人员和其他艇上人员数量及健康状况；

（四）依法应当向检验检疫机构申报并接受检疫的动植物、动植物产品和其他检疫物。

**第七条** 艇方或者其代理人应当在游艇到达检疫地点前12小时将确定到达的日期和时间通知检验检疫机构。

**第八条** 无重大疫病疫情时，艇方或者其代理人可以向检验检疫机构申请电讯检疫，并提供《交通工具卫生证书》、《船舶免予卫生控制措施证书/船舶卫生控制措施证书》。

未持有上述证书的，检验检疫机构可以先予实施电讯检疫，艇方或者其代理人在游艇抵达检疫地点后应当申请补办。

第九条 有下列情形之一的游艇，艇方或者其代理人应当主动向检验检疫机构报告，由检验检疫机构在检疫锚地或者检验检疫机构指定的地点实施检疫：

（一）来自受染地区的；

（二）来自动植物疫区，国家有明确要求的；

（三）有受染病人、疑似受染病人，或者有人非因意外伤害而死亡并死因不明的；

（四）发现有啮齿动物异常死亡的。

第十条 除实施电讯检疫的以及本办法第九条规定的检疫以外的其他游艇，由检验检疫机构在口岸开放码头或者经检验检疫机构同意的游艇停泊水域或者码头实施靠泊检疫。

需要办理口岸临时开放手续的，按照相关规定执行。

第十一条 受入境检疫的游艇应当按照规定悬挂检疫信号等候查验，在检疫完毕并签发《船舶入境检疫证书》后，方可解除检疫信号、上下人员、装卸行李等物品。

不具备悬挂检疫信号条件的，入境时应当在检疫地点等候查验，并尽早通知检验检疫机构实施检疫。

第十二条 办理入境检疫手续时，艇方或者其代理人应当向检验检疫机构提交《出/入境游艇检疫总申报单》、

《船舶免予卫生控制措施证书/船舶卫生控制措施证书》、游艇操作人员及随艇人员名单等相关资料,必要时提供游艇航行等相关记录。来自黄热病疫区的,还应当提供艇上人员《预防接种证书》。

不能提供《船舶免予卫生控制措施证书/船舶卫生控制措施证书》的,艇方或者其代理人在游艇入境后应当向检验检疫机构申请补办。

**第十三条** 检验检疫机构依法对入境游艇上的受染病人实施隔离,对疑似受染病人实施不超过受染传染病潜伏期的留验或者就地诊验。

**第十四条** 入境游艇有下列情形之一的,应当实施检疫处理:

(一)来自受染地区的;

(二)被受染病人、疑似受染病人污染的;

(三)发现有与人类健康有关的医学媒介生物,超过国家卫生标准的;

(四)发现有动物一类、二类传染病、寄生虫病或者进境植物检疫性有害生物的。

**第十五条** 入境游艇在中国境内停留期间,艇上人员不得将所装载的动植物、动植物产品和其他检疫物带离游艇;需要带离时,应当向检验检疫机构报检,相关程序及要求按照《出入境人员携带物检疫管理办法》及其他法律法规的相关规定执行。

游艇上装载有禁止进境的动植物、动植物产品和其他检疫物的,检验检疫机构应当做封存或者销毁处理。

第十六条 携带犬、猫(以下简称宠物)入境的,每人每次限带1只,携带人应当向检验检疫机构提供输出国家或者地区官方动物检疫机构出具的有效检疫证书和疫苗接种证书。宠物应当具有芯片或者其他有效身份证明。

第十七条 来自非狂犬病发生国家或者地区的宠物,经查验证书符合要求且现场检疫合格的,可以办理宠物入境随行手续。

来自狂犬病发生国家或者地区的宠物,应当在检验检疫机构指定的隔离场所隔离30天。

工作犬,如导盲犬、搜救犬等,携带人提供相应证明且现场检疫合格的,可以免于隔离检疫。

检验检疫机构对隔离检疫的宠物实行监督检查。

第十八条 入境宠物有下列情形之一的,禁止带离游艇:

(一)入境宠物无输出国家或者地区官方动物检疫机构出具的有效检疫证书和疫苗接种证书的;

(二)数量超过限额的;

(三)现场检疫不合格的。

第十九条 入境游艇经检疫查验合格的,由检验检疫机构签发《船舶入境检疫证书》等证单。

## 第三章　出境检疫

**第二十条**　游艇出境时,应当在出境 3 小时前向出境口岸检验检疫机构申报并办理出境检疫手续。办理出境检疫手续后出现人员变动或者其他特殊情况 24 小时内不能出境的,须重新办理。

游艇在入境口岸停留不足 24 小时出境的,经检验检疫机构同意,在办理入境手续时,可以同时办理出境手续。

**第二十一条**　办理出境检疫手续时,艇方或者其代理人应当向检验检疫机构提交《出/入境游艇检疫总申报单》、游艇操作人员及随艇人员名单等有关资料。入境时已提交且无变动的,经艇方或者其代理人书面声明,可以免予提供。

**第二十二条**　出境游艇经检疫查验合格的,由检验检疫机构签发《交通工具出境卫生检疫证书》等证单。

## 第四章　监督管理

**第二十三条**　游艇入境后,发现受染病人或者突发公共卫生事件,或者有人非因意外伤害而死亡并死因不明的,艇方或者其代理人应当及时向到达的口岸检验检疫机构报告,接受临时检疫。

**第二十四条** 游艇在境内航行、停留期间,不得擅自启封、动用检验检疫机构在艇上封存的物品。

游艇上的生活垃圾、泔水、动植物性废弃物等,艇方应当放置于密封的容器中,在离艇前应当实施必要的检疫处理。

**第二十五条** 检验检疫机构对游艇实施卫生监督,对卫生状况不良和可能导致传染病传播或者检疫性有害生物传播扩散的因素提出改进意见,并监督指导采取必要的检疫处理措施。

**第二十六条** 检验检疫机构对游艇专用停泊水域或者码头、游艇俱乐部实施卫生监督,游艇俱乐部和艇方或者其代理人应当予以配合。

**第二十七条** 游艇停泊水域或者码头,满足下列条件的,经检验检疫机构同意,可以在该水域或者码头实施检疫:

(一)具备管理和回收游艇废弃物、垃圾等的能力;

(二)具备对废弃物、垃圾等进行无害化处理的能力;

(三)具备相关的口岸检验检疫设施,满足检验检疫机构查验和检疫处理的需求。

**第二十八条** 游艇在境内停留期间发生传染病疫情

或者突发公共卫生事件等,检验检疫机构应当及时启动应急预案,科学应对,妥善处置,防止疫病疫情扩散传播。

**第二十九条** 检验检疫机构根据需要可以在游艇码头等场所设立工作点,实行驻点服务。

# 第五章 法律责任

**第三十条** 有下列违法行为之一的,由检验检疫机构处以警告或者100元以上5000元以下的罚款:

(一)入境、出境的游艇,在入境检疫之前或者在出境检疫之后,擅自上下人员,装卸行李、货物等物品的;

(二)入境、出境的游艇拒绝接受检疫或者抵制卫生监督,拒不接受检疫处理的;

(三)伪造或者涂改卫生检疫证单的;

(四)瞒报携带禁止进境的微生物、人体组织、生物制品、血液及其制品或者其他可能引起传染病传播的动物和物品的;

(五)携带动植物、动植物产品和其他检疫物入境,未依法办理检疫审批手续或者未按照检疫审批的规定执行的。

**第三十一条** 有下列违法行为之一的,由检验检疫机构处以1000元以上1万元以下的罚款:

（一）未经检疫或者未经检疫合格的入境、出境游艇，擅自离开检疫地点，逃避查验的；

（二）隐瞒疫情或者伪造情节的；

（三）未实施检疫处理，擅自排放压舱水，移下垃圾、污物等物品的；

（四）未实施检疫处理，擅自移运尸体、骸骨的。

第三十二条　未经检疫查验，从游艇上移下传染病病人造成传染病传播危险的，由检验检疫机构处以5000元以上3万元以下的罚款。

第三十三条　有下列违法行为之一的，由检验检疫机构处以3000元以上3万元以下的罚款：

（一）未经检验检疫机构许可擅自将随艇进境、过境动植物、动植物产品和其他检疫物卸离游艇或者运递的；

（二）擅自调离或者处理在检验检疫机构指定的隔离场所中隔离检疫的动植物的；

（三）擅自开拆、损毁检验检疫封识或者标志的；

（四）擅自抛弃随艇过境的动物尸体、排泄物、铺垫材料或者其他废弃物，或者未按规定处理游艇上的泔水、动植物性废弃物的；

（五）艇上人员违反本办法规定，携带无官方动物检疫证书，或者检疫发现有疫病疫情的宠物上岸的。

第三十四条　艇上人员有其他应当申报而未申报，或者申报的内容与实际不符的,由检验检疫机构处以警告或者5000元以下的罚款。

**第三十五条** 出入境人员拒绝、阻碍检验检疫机构及其工作人员依法执行职务的,依法移送有关部门处理。

**第三十六条** 受行政处罚的当事人应当在出境前履行检验检疫机构作出的行政处罚决定。当事人向指定的银行缴纳罚款确有困难,经当事人提出,检验检疫机构及其执法人员可以当场收缴罚款。当场收缴罚款的,必须向当事人出具罚款收据。

执法人员当场收缴的罚款,应当自收缴罚款之日起2日内,交至行政机关;在水上当场收缴的罚款,应当自抵岸之日起2日内交至行政机关;行政机关应当在2日内将罚款缴付指定的银行。

**第三十七条** 检验检疫机构工作人员应当秉公执法、忠于职守,不得滥用职权、玩忽职守、徇私舞弊;违法失职的,依法追究责任。

# 第六章 附 则

**第三十八条** 本办法所称:

"游艇"仅限于用于游览观光、休闲娱乐等活动的具备机械推进动力装置的船舶。

"艇方"是指游艇所有人或者其使用人。

"艇上人员"包括游艇上的操作人员以及乘坐游艇的所有人员。

"游艇俱乐部"包括为出入境游艇提供游艇靠泊、保管及使用服务的依法成立的游艇俱乐部、游艇会以及其他组织。

"受染"是指受到感染或者污染(包括核放射、生物、化学因子),或者携带感染源或者污染源,包括携带医学媒介生物和宿主,可能引起国际关注的传染病或者构成其他严重公共卫生危害的。

"受染嫌疑"是指检验检疫机构认为已经暴露于或者可能暴露于严重公共卫生危害,并且有可能成为传染源或者污染源。

"受染人(物)"是指受到感染或者污染或者携带感染源或者污染源以至于构成公共卫生风险的人员、宠物、行李、物品、游艇等。

"受染地区"是指需采取卫生措施的特定地理区域。

第三十九条 经国家质检总局批准,其他地区出入境游艇检疫监督管理工作可以参照本办法执行。

第四十条 本办法由国家质检总局负责解释。

第四十一条 本办法自2013年8月1日起施行。

# Contents

Decree of General Administration of Quality Supervision, Inspection and Quarantine of the People's Republic of China
(2013 No. 153) ·················· 17

Administrative Measures on Quarantine of Entry-Exit Yachts of Hainan Province ··· 19
Chapter Ⅰ　General Provisions ·················· 19
Chapter Ⅱ　Entry Quarantine ·················· 21
Chapter Ⅲ　Exit Quarantine ·················· 29
Chapter Ⅳ　Supervision and Administration ·········· 31
Chapter Ⅴ　Legal Liabilities ·················· 34
Chapter Ⅵ　Supplementary Provisions ·················· 39

In case of any discrepancies between the Chinese version and the English version, the Chinese version shall prevail.

# Decree of General Administration of Quality Supervision, Inspection and Quarantine of the People's Republic of China

## No. 153

The *Administrative Measures on Quarantine of Entry-Exit Yachts of Hainan Province* as reviewed and adopted at the ministerial meeting of the General Administration of Quality Supervision, Inspection and Quarantine of the People's Republic of China on April 23, 2013, are hereby promulgated and shall enter into force as of August 1, 2013.

Minister  *Zhi Shuping*

June 5, 2013

# Administrative Measures on Quarantine of Entry-Exit Yachts of Hainan Province

## Chapter I  General Provisions

**Article 1**  For the purpose of preventing epidemics and diseases from spreading into or out of the territory of People's Republic of China and regulating the quarantine of entry-exit yachts of Hainan Province, these Measures are formulated in accordance with the laws and regulations such as the *Frontier Health and Quarantine Law of the People's Republic of China* and the specific rules for its implementation, the *Law of the People's Republic of China on the Entry and Exit Animal and Plant Quarantine* and the regulations for its implementation, the *International Health Regulation*, as well as the related provisions of the State Council.

**Article 2**  These Measures shall apply to the quarantine, supervision and administration of the yachts entering or exiting the territory of the People's Republic of China in Hainan Province.

**Article 3**  The General Administration of Quality Supervision, Inspection and Quarantine (hereinafter referred to as "AQSIQ") takes principal charge of the supervision and administration of the quarantine of entry-exit yachts throughout the country.

The entry-exit inspection and quarantine authorities established by AQSIQ in Hainan Province (hereinafter referred to as "the inspection and quarantine authorities") are responsible for the quarantine of entry-exit yachts and its supervision and administration in Hainan Province.

**Article 4**  The quarantine, supervision and administration of the entry-exit yachts in Hainan Province shall follow the principles of first try, effective supervision and administration, simplified procedures, as well as convenience and efficiency.

## Chapter II    Entry Quarantine

**Article 5**    The entry yacht shall be subjected to quarantine at the first port of arrival.

The inspection and quarantine authority may conduct quarantine on the entry yacht by telecommunication, and/or quarantine at anchorage, at berth or on board during voyage.

**Article 6**    Before the yacht arrives at the port, the yacht party or its agent shall declare the following information to the inspection and quarantine authority of the entry port:
(1) Name and nationality of the yacht and the estimated date and time of arrival at the quarantine place;

(2) Port of departure and port of the last call;

(3) The number of yacht operators and other people on board as well as their health conditions;

(4) Animals and plants, their products and other quarantine objects that shall be declared to and quarantined by the inspection and quarantine authority in accordance with law.

**Article 7** The yacht party or its agent shall inform the inspection and quarantine authority of the confirmed date and time of arrival 12 hours before the yacht arrives at the quarantine place.

**Article 8** When there are no serious epidemics and diseases, the yacht party or its agent may apply for quarantine by telecommunication to the inspection and quarantine authority and should provide Health Quarantine Certificate for Conveyance and Ship Sanitation Control Exemption Certificate / Ship Sanitation Control Certificate.

In case of unavailability of the above-mentioned certificates, the inspection and quarantine authority may implement quarantine by telecommunication first, and the yacht party or its agent shall submit the post-application for such certificates after the yacht arrives at the quarantine place.

**Article 9** In case of any of the following circumstances, the yacht party or its agent shall take the initiative in reporting to the inspection and quarantine authority which shall implement quarantine at the quarantine anchorage or other places designated by the inspection and quarantine authority:

(1) The yacht comes from a contaminated area;

(2) The yacht comes from an animal and plant epidemic area, for which quarantine is explicitly required by the State;

(3) There are quarantinable epidemic victims, quarantinable epidemic suspects, or a person dies from an unidentified cause other than accidental injuries;

(4) Abnormal death of rodent is found.

**Article 10** Except the yachts subject to quarantine by

telecommunication and quarantine specified in Article 9 of these Measures, the inspection and quarantine authority shall conduct quarantine at an open wharf or in a yacht mooring water area or at a wharf approved by the inspection and quarantine authority.

The procedure for temporary port opening, if required, shall be carried out in accordance with relevant provisions.

**Article 11** The yacht subject to entry quarantine shall hang a quarantine signal and wait for inspection in accordance with the provisions. Removal of the quarantine signal, embarking or disembarking, and/or loading or unloading luggage and other articles are not allowed until the quarantine is completed and a Free Pratique is issued.

The yacht without the equipment of hanging a quarantine signal shall wait for inspection in the quarantine place at the time of entry, and inform the inspection and quarantine authority to implement quarantine as early as possible.

**Article 12** When going through the entry quarantine procedures, the yacht party or its agent shall submit to the inspection and quarantine authority General Declaration for Entry-Exit Yacht Quarantine, Ship Sanitation Control Exemption Certificate / Ship Sanitation Control Certificate, a name list of yacht operators and people on board and other relevant documents, and such records as a yacht log book if necessary. If the yacht comes from an epidemic area contaminated by yellow fever, the Certificate of Vaccination or Prophylaxis of the people on board shall also be provided.

In case of unavailability of Ship Sanitation Control Exemption Certificate / Ship Sanitation Control Certificate, the yacht party or its agent shall submit the post-application for such certificates to the inspection and quarantine authority after entry of the yacht.

**Article 13** Inspection and quarantine authorities shall implement isolation of quarantinable epidemic victims on the entry yachts in accordance with the law. For quarantinable epidemic suspects, inspection and quarantine authorities shall implement check-up detention with duration not longer than the latent period of the contaminating epidemic, or conduct on-site clinical check-up.

**Article 14** In case of any of the following circumstances, the entry yacht shall be subjected to quarantine treatment:

(1) The yacht comes from a contaminated area;

(2) The yacht is contaminated by quarantinable epidemic victims or quarantinable epidemic suspects;

(3) The medical vectors relating to human health exceed the limit specified in the national health standards;

(4) Animal infectious or parasitic diseases Class A or Class B or entry plant quarantine pests are found.

**Article 15** During stay of an entry yacht within the territory, the people on board shall not take away the animals and plants, their products and other quarantine objects on board from the yacht. If such take-away is requested, one must apply for the inspection to the inspection and quarantine authority, carry out the procedures and meet the requirements in accordance with the provisions of the *Administrative Measures on Quarantine of Articles Carried by Entry and Exit Passengers* and other related laws and regulations.

Where a yacht is loaded with entry-prohibited animals and plants, their products and other quarantine objects, inspection and quarantine authorities shall seal or destroy them.

**Article 16** Whoever carries dogs or cats (hereinafter referred to as "the pets") into the territory, shall be limited to carrying only one per person each time and submit to the inspection and quarantine authority the valid quarantine certificate and the vaccination certificate issued by the official animal quarantine authority of the exporting country or region. The pets shall have microchips or other valid identity certifications.

**Article 17** The pets from the rabies-free countries or regions may go through accompanying pet entry procedures if their certificates meet the requirements and they have passed on-site quarantine.

The pets from the rabies-endemic countries or regions are subjected to isolation quarantine for a period of 30 days at the isolation area designated by the inspection and quarantine authorities.

Working dogs, such as guide dogs, search and rescue dogs, etc., may be exempted from the isolation quarantine upon presentation of the relevant certificates by the carrier and after they have passed on-site quarantine.

Inspection and quarantine authorities shall perform observation and examination on the pets isolated for quarantine.

**Article 18** In case of any of the following circumstances, the entry pets shall not be taken away from the yacht:

(1) There are no valid quarantine certificates and vaccination certificates issued by official animal quarantine authorities of the exporting countries or regions for entry pets;

(2) The quantitative limit of pets is exceeded;

(3) The pets fail to pass on-site quarantine.

**Article 19** Where the entry yacht has passed quarantine inspection, the inspection and quarantine authority shall issue a Free Pratique and other documents.

## Chapter Ⅲ  Exit Quarantine

**Article 20** The yacht party or its agent shall apply for the inspection to the inspection and quarantine authority of the exit port and go through the exit quarantine procedures at least 3 hours before the yacht exits. The yacht party or its agent shall reapply for the inspection if, after the completion of the exit quarantine procedures, any special circumstance occurs that prevents the yacht from departing within 24 hours or any personnel change has happened.

Where the yacht stays in the port of entry less than 24 hours before exit, it may go through exit procedures along with entry procedures upon approval of the inspection and quarantine authority.

**Article 21** While going through exit procedures, the yacht party or its agent shall submit to the inspection and quarantine authority the General Declaration for Entry-Exit Yacht Quarantine, the name list of yacht operators and people on board, as well as other relevant documents. If they have been submitted at the time of entry and no modifications occur hereafter, such documents may be exempted from submission upon written declaration by the yacht party or its agent.

**Article 22** Where an exit yacht has passed quarantine inspection, the inspection and quarantine authority shall issue the Health Quarantine Certificate for Departure of Conveyance and other documents.

## Chapter Ⅳ  Supervision and Administration

**Article 23**  Where quarantinable epidemic victims are found, or a public health emergency occurs, or a person dies from an unidentified cause other than accidental injuries after entry of a yacht, the yacht party or its agent shall make a timely report to the inspection and quarantine authority of the port of arrival and accept temporary quarantine.

**Article 24**  Without authorization, on-board articles sealed by the inspection and quarantine authority shall not be unsealed or used during navigation and stay of a yacht within the territory.

The on-board garbage, swills and wastes of animal or plant nature shall be kept in sealed containers by the yacht party and undergo necessary quarantine treatment before leaving the yacht.

**Article 25**  The inspection and quarantine authorities implement sanitary control on yachts, give improvement suggestions on poor sanitary conditions and the factors that may possibly cause the transmission of infectious diseases or the spread and diffusion of quarantine pests, and supervise and guide the adoption of necessary quarantine treatment measures.

**Article 26** The inspection and quarantine authorities implement sanitary control on the mooring water areas or wharves exclusively used for yachts as well as yacht clubs. Yacht clubs and the yacht party or its agent shall be cooperative in this regard.

**Article 27** When the yacht mooring water area or a wharf meets the following conditions and upon approval of the inspection and quarantine authority, quarantine may be conducted in the said areas:

(1) It has the capacity to manage and collect yacht wastes, garbage, etc. ;

(2) It has the capacity to conduct bio-safety treatment of

wastes and garbage;

(3) It is equipped with the relevant port inspection and quarantine facilities and meets the requirements of the inspection and quarantine authority for inspection and quarantine treatment.

**Article 28**　In the event that the epidemic of an infectious disease or a public health emergency occurs during the stay of a yacht within the territory, the inspection and quarantine authority shall initiate the contingency plan in time, cope with the event scientifically, handle it properly and prevent the spread and diffusion of the epidemics and diseases.

**Article 29**　The inspection and quarantine authority, where necessary, may set up working points at such places as yacht wharves to provide regular services at those points.

## Chapter V  Legal Liabilities

**Article 30**  Whoever, in violation of law, commits any of the following acts shall be given a warning or imposed a fine of not less than 100 yuan but not more than 5,000 yuan by the inspection and quarantine authority:

(1) Without authorization, embarking or disembarking, and/or loading or unloading luggage, goods and other articles from an entry or exit yacht before entry quarantine or after exit quarantine;

(2) Refusing to accept the quarantine inspection or resisting sanitary control or rejecting quarantine treatment by an entry or exit yacht;

(3) Forging or altering health and quarantine certificates and documents;

(4) Concealment in declaring of carrying such articles as microzoaria, human tissue, biologicals, blood and hemo-

products which are prohibited from entering into the territory or other animals and objects which may cause the spread of epidemic diseases;

(5) Carrying animals and plants, their products and other quarantine objects into the territory without going through formalities for examination and approval of quarantine inspection in accordance with law or failing to follow the provisions on examination and approval of quarantine inspection.

**Article 31**  Whoever, in violation of law, commits any of the following acts shall be imposed a fine of not less than 1000 yuan but not more than 10,000 yuan by the inspection and quarantine authority:

(1) Without authorization, leaving the quarantine place to evade inspection for an entry or exit yacht without quarantine or failing the quarantine;

(2) Concealing the epidemics or falsifying the situation;

(3) Without authorization, discharging ballast water and unloading garbage, dirt and other articles with no quarantine treatment;

(4) Without authorization, removing or transporting corpses or human remains with no quarantine treatment.

**Article 32**　Where patients with infectious diseases are removed from a yacht without quarantine inspection, which causes the risk of transmission of the infectious diseases, a fine of not less than 5,000 yuan and not more than 30,000 yuan shall be imposed by the inspection and quarantine authority.

**Article 33**　Whoever, in violation of law, commits any of the following acts shall be imposed a fine of not less than 3,000 yuan but not more than 30,000 yuan by the inspection and quarantine authority:

(1) Without the permission of the inspection and quarantine authorities, unloading animals or plants, their products or other quarantine objects from the yacht entering or

transiting the territory, or transporting or delivering the above articles;

(2) Without permission, transferring or disposing of animals and plants subject to isolation quarantine in isolated areas designated by the inspection and quarantine authorities;

(3) Without authorization, removing or damaging the seals or marks for inspection and quarantine;

(4) Without authorization, casting away dead body of animals, excrements, bedding materials or other wastes on the yacht transiting the territory, or disposing of, not in accordance with the provisions, the swills and wastes of animal or plant nature of the yacht;

(5) People on board, in violation of the provisions of these Measures, carrying ashore the pets without official animal quarantine certificates or the pets found to have an epidemic disease during quarantine.

**Article 34** Where the people on board subject to declaration have not made the declaration or the declaration is inconsistent with the actual situations, they shall be issued a warning or imposed a fine of not more than 5,000 yuan by the inspection and quarantine authority.

**Article 35** Entry-Exit passengers refusing or obstructing the inspection and quarantine authorities and their staff from performing their official duties shall be transferred to and handled by the relevant authorities in accordance with law.

**Article 36** The parties subject to administrative penalty shall carry out the decisions on administrative penalty before leaving the territory. If it is really difficult for the parties to pay the fines to the bank as designated, the inspection and quarantine authority and its law-enforcing officers may, upon the request of the parties, collect the fines on the spot. Where fines are collected on the spot, the parties shall be given receipts for the fines.

Fines collected by law-enforcing officers on the spot shall

be turned over to the administrative organs within 2 days from the date the fines are collected. Fines collected on the spot on water shall be turned over to the administrative organs within 2 days from the date of landing. The administrative organs shall deliver the fines over to the banks as designated within 2 days.

**Article 37** Any staff of inspection and quarantine authorities shall enforce law impartially, perform duties faithfully and shall not abuse their powers, neglect their duties or commit illegalities for personal interests; those who violate the law or fail to perform their duties, shall be investigated for liabilities in accordance with law.

## Chapter Ⅵ Supplementary Provisions

**Article 38** In these Measures:
"Yachts" are limited to the ships intended for activities such as sightseeing, leisure and recreation, and equipped with mechanically propelled power installations.

"Yacht party" refers to the owner or user of a yacht.

"People on board" includes all the persons on a yacht, i. e. the operators and passengers of the yacht.

"Yacht clubs" includes yacht clubs and other organizations established in accordance with law to provide mooring, safekeeping and usage services for entry-exit yachts.

"Contaminated" refers to being infected or contaminated (nuclear radiation, biological and chemical factors inclusive), or carrying sources of infection or contamination (including medical vectors and reservoirs), which may possibly induce infectious diseases of international concerns or constitute other serious public hazards.

"Quarantinable epidemic suspects" refers to the objects that the inspection and quarantine authority considers to have been exposed or might be exposed to serious public health hazards and may become sources of infection or contamination.

"Quarantinable epidemic victims (objects)" refers to the people, the pets, luggage, articles, yachts, etc. that are infected or contaminated or carry sources of infection or contamination, which may subsequently constitute public health risks.

"Contaminated area" refers to a specific geographic area that needs taking sanitary measures.

**Article 39** Subject to the approval of AQSIQ, the quarantine, supervision and administration on entry-exit yachts in other regions may be implemented with reference to these Measures.

**Article 40** These Measures are interpreted by AQSIQ.

**Article 41** These Measures shall enter into force as of August 1, 2013.